CRY LEARN ADJUST FiGHT AND REPEAT!

MARQUITA GOODLUCK

Cover art and design by Theresa A. Stites

For Tilly,

You were such an amazing human being.
You always exuded light, energy, and
positivity in every situation.
I will always keep you in my heart.
You will be forever missed.

I love you.

CONTENTS

INTRODUCTION

I am sure you have seen her. She is the woman in the waiting room. The one flooding your social media time-line with positivity. The woman with a huge support system. She is the one participating in a Breast Cancer walk. The one who loses friends to Breast Cancer often, but still brave enough to get up and fight. The one who has lost almost everything that made her a woman, yet still shows up with style. The one who has mastered to stay happy in spite of it all. She seems completely fearless. Everyone is amazed by all of her accomplishments. You look at her and wonder how can I be like her? Why am I not this positive? Where does she get this strength from? You can barely say the words " I have Breast Cancer" out loud, let alone share it with the world and jump into warrior mode. You are struggling to see your future, which seems so blocked by a new Breast Cancer diagnosis. Just coming to terms with the entire process has been over-whelming. You tell yourself, I can't wait to skip to that part! When will I reach that point in my journey! Is it even possible?

Well, I am here to tell you that it is very possible! You can and will gain control of your life again! Your life will be different than you could ever imagine, but it will go on. You will learn to live a more meaningful life. You will treasure every moment and make every moment count. I know this, because I was you! I have been where you are! I was diagnosed with Breast Cancer at 35 and it truly rocked my world. It changed everything.

On August 17, 2017, I was diagnosed with Breast Cancer. What started out as a simple lump, completely altered my life. My life as I knew it came to a halt. Doctor visit after doctor visit, advice after advice, my life slowly became unrecognizable. Enraged with my diagnosis, all my hopes, goals, and dreams slowly disappeared. Dealing with months of chemotherapy and radiation, I felt powerless and defeated. It was almost as if my future was blocked. Overwhelmed with this neverending feeling of defeat, I knew that I had to save myself. I knew that the doctors would handle my treatment plan but it was up to me to control my mental state. In an effort to gain control, I immediately jumped in survivor mode. I didn't know if I could find happiness or positivity, but I knew that I had fight in me! I knew that I was determined to win. After my doctors created a treatment plan for me, I too, created a treatment plan for me. One that I would do on my end, to win this battle.

I started connecting with other Breast Cancer survivors, educating myself, and controlling the controllables. I couldn't control the Cancer, side effects, nor the treatment, but, I could control how I handled it. So I took on Breast Cancer bit by bit. I handled every treatment and side effect one problem at a time. In the midst of my journey, I created my motto which would see me through it all: CRY, LEARN, ADJUST, FIGHT & REPEAT. This motto has helped me during my journey and continues to help me to this day. Every treatment, appointment, or side effect was so scary. But by applying my mantra: CRY, LEARN, ADJUST, FIGHT & REPEAT, I learned that the TEARS would relieve my soul, rage, and anger. The RESEARCH, would equip me with the tools to fight.

The ACCEPTANCE of change, would help me to adjust to my situation and EMPOWER me to fight, and I would do this over and over again.

*I*n this book, I will highlight the common fears and issues that women may face or struggle with during their Breast Cancer journey and provide ways to get through it. I am not a doctor and this book is not a medical guide. It is my testament. In an effort to inspire women to fight and keep their strength, I will share my journey. Hopefully, by the end of this book, you too will find the strength to

CRY, LEARN, ADJUST, FIGHT, AND REPEAT!

-M.Goodluck

"Life is not measured by the number of breaths we take, but by the moments that take our breath away."

- Maya Angelou

Chapter 1

HELLO LUMP!

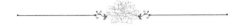

What should I do? Will I die? How will I tell my family?

Like most women who are diagnosed under the age of 40, I thought that Breast Cancer was an older woman's struggle. Never did I imagine that I would be diagnosed with this horrible disease. I found my lump by doing a self-exam. Immediately when I felt it, I knew something was not quite right. But never did I imagine it was Cancer. I was convinced that I was not the typical patient. I shopped at Whole Foods, ate healthy, took vitamins, breastfed my kids, and was pretty healthy. In my mind, I thought this lump must be a cyst....there is no way it's Breast Cancer. But after a two mammograms, two biopsies, and a call from my doctor, I was injected head first into the world of Breast Cancer. I was diagnosed with stage two Invasive Ductal Carcinoma. My treatment plan consisted of 4 rounds of chemotherapy, a bilateral mastectomy, and 25 rounds of radiation, and one year of my life.

What should I do?

When I was initially diagnosed my first fear was what should I do? How can I win in this situation? All my life I was used to finding a solution. Vulnerability wasn't a part of my DNA. I was someone who was always a fighter or problem solver. I first thought to myself you will beat this.

You will take herbs and vitamins. You got this! There is no way that this will be how your story will end. I was very positive from the start but little by little my positivity started to diminish. When they said I would have to do chemo, I was saddened but then I got used to the idea, then they said I needed a mastectomy, I was frightened, then I got over it, by the time they told me I needed radiation and physical therapy, I started to lose my faith and hope. I couldn't understand why nothing seemed to be going my way.

As if a Cancer diagnosis wasn't enough, I felt that the mental battle was way more cruel. Every time I convinced myself that I was strong enough to win, the more appointments I had, the more information I received, the more overwhelmed I became. During this process is when I learned that I was not in control. I could not control the doctors, the side effects of my treatment, and my body during treatment. There was no going around it. I had to go through it all. I had to accept help and be willing to have my life placed on hold. I had to accept this temporary change. I knew I could only focus on controlling the controllables.

When you are in the planning or research stage, it can be difficult to find any peace. One of the techniques I started to apply to my journey was acceptance. Of course acceptance sounds difficult to accomplish right away, but I believe that the faster you learn to accept a situation, the better you can deal with a situation. There are no surprises. So, I would thoroughly research certain treatments,

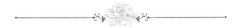
side effects and remedies. By getting a clear understanding of what needs to be done and what will most likely happen after, I was able to gain control over my mental state. I told myself that my life would be uncomfortable for a year, but I would win this battle and come out on top.

Build a great team

For the fight of your life, it's only suitable for you to get an all-star team of doctors and the only way to accomplish that is through research, references from other doctors, and your intuition. Intuition is everything when fighting Breast Cancer! I believe that to find your correct path you have to be intuitive and follow your gut feelings. When dealing with Breast Cancer, your internal feelings are great indicators to help you make good decisions. You will be bombarded with so many talented doctors, that it will be difficult to see what doctor will work for you. I found that after research, the only thing that helped me to select my doctors was my heart and gut feelings. I chose who spoke to my spirit, who was willing to educate, whoever was experienced and knowledgeable, and someone with great energy.

I knew I couldn't control my journey completely, but I knew I could choose great people to help me save my life. So my first step in my journey, was to build a great team. One thing I learned in my journey is that great doctors recommend other great doctors and this helped me on my journey. My radiologist referred me to my breast surgeon, my breast surgeon referred me to my plastic surgeon, and my breast surgeon referred me to my oncologist, and my plastic surgeon referred me to my radiation oncologist. Being directed to very successful and caring doctors in my area, gave me a sense of peace. I researched and researched and found some of the best Cancer centers in my area. I met with doctors and only chose the ones who spoke to my spirit. To me the ideal doctor is one that has ample experience, is willing to educate, has patience, availability, and empathy. The key to choosing doctors in this journey is to choose doctors that are all on the same page. It's important to choose doctors who all agree with the treatment plan you have chosen, only then will you feel at ease. Some of your fears will diminish when you know your life is in trusted hands. Since these doctors specialized in Breast Cancer, they were very knowledge-able. It helped to ease my fear of dying and being vulnera-ble. My confidence in their skills, diminished stress and anxiety. We were all on the same page and all focusing on the same goal. I felt like I was gaining control of the situation by making a dream team that would get me through this journey.

Will I die?

It would be remiss of me to not address the biggest fear, death. There are so many images of Breast Cancer survivors thriving and surviving, but the reality is that some actually don't win their battle. This was and still is a constant fear of mine. But, I find that no Breast Cancer is the same, everyone is different and has different treatment plans. I believe you can't worry about the future, you should focus on the fight. By changing your life and controlling your mental state, you can win. Many women survive and are thriving. I believe it's best to flip your fear of death by transforming it more into a bucket list. In order to be up for a battle, I had to transform my thought process. Instead of focusing on dying, I focused on the business of living. For me, this meant that the fear of death was always there, so I should take every chance or opportunity to live my best life. I learned to live a more free and adventurous life. I understood the value in a day, month, and year!! All my fears of dying I conquered by making an effort to erase fear in other areas of my life. Whatever I wanted to do or used to be to scared to do, I did.

Since my diagnosis, I treasure every moment. Since I know that death is a possibility, I have decided to live a life full of positivity, adventure, love, and fun. While I was in chemo, I created a bucket list for my life and as soon as treatment was over I started to work on accomplishing things off of my bucket list. I told myself to be fearless and live. I also, decided from the start to control my mental state, because I knew that my mental state played a huge part in my journey. So I would control, what I watched or read. I was only about positivity. I stopped worrying about every possible side effect and I stopped googling Breast Cancer statistics. I even found that Breast Cancer forums, although extremely helpful, can be damaging to your mental state. I realize I had to minimize how much time I spent on the forums. To me, the forums made me feel as if everyone was dying or unsuccessful on their journey. I had to realize that that wasn't a correct representation of all Breast Cancer survivors, it just felt like everyone was dying because they are all gathered together in one place, but in reality, some women actually survive. This belief made it easier for me to be on the forums. I realized that although it's sad to see someone lose their battle, others are winning, and maybe I would be one of the ones that win.

How will I tell my family?

When I first started my journey, I went to all my appointments in secret. Other than my husband, no one knew what was going on. Being a mother of three, telling my kids was my biggest fear. I just didn't know how to explain it and how they would survive with knowing my diagnosis. I really felt that their little broken hearts would crush me and I would for sure, lose my fight. This is the fear that kept me up at night. More than dying, more than the treatment, I feared stealing their innocence and happiness by telling them of my reality. My first plan was to keep it a secret as long as I could, but after talking to my oncologist, I realize that wasn't possible. It was foolish of me to think I could take on a huge journey without telling them. But with the help of my oncologist, I found the right tone and set of words to tell them. My children were the ages of 7,9, and 12. I sat them down one day and simply told them that, I have Breast Cancer, it's very early, but I have to take care of it now so I don't have to worry about it later. Surprisingly, this eased their fears. Knowing that I wasn't in any pain but I was just preventing the cancer cells from growing. I also told my children that at some point I may look sick or exhausted, but that will be from the chemo I will be taking. I have learned that the key to telling children is to be completely honest but also keep a positive attitude. They will mimic your energy. If you take it on as a fighter, then they will fight to be strong for you. By being upfront with your kids and telling them what to expect, you can help them deal with your treatment plan. When I told my children, I made a vow to myself to not let it affect our entire life. I attempted to live the life I normally lived, just with a few changes.

Dealing with family

Ugh, one of the things I truly hated in my journey, is the ignorance of some family and friends. Though no fault of their own, many of my conversations were damaging to my mental state. When family or friends initially heard of my diagnosis, they would immediately say things like:

"You will be fine, I know someone who had it and they just took it out"

" My friend had the same cancer and she died"

"My friend had Chemo and her cancer still came back"

"I could never do Chemotherapy"

"I don't believe in Chemo."

"I don't understand why you have to do chemo and a mastectomy, get a second opinion."

"You can treat it with lemons."

"You shouldn't get implants"

"You never know how strong you are, I think you can live without breasts. You shouldn't get reconstruction."

"Why are your doctors being so aggressive?"

"Why are you telling people?"

"Implants are unsafe."

"You know some people die from the Chemo alone."

Although, I forgive them for all their ignorant comments, I just chucked it up to they just didn't know. However, I learned very quickly the importance of keeping parts of my treatment and journey a secret. I knew that everyone wasn't ready to receive my treatment plans and lack the knowledge to understand it. Therefore, I kept parts of my treatment private. If there was a procedure I was worried about, I would only confide in a few people who I knew could handle it. I knew that there were no benefits to telling someone who would just scare me. So I decided to share more in depth details of my treatment plan with a select few. I would let most people know I was in treatment, but I never discussed issues or details. I found that their statements bothered me deeply and made me question my decisions. I learn that in order to beat this disease, you have to be confident in your decisions and treatments. There is no room for toxic people or naysayers. If you have these type of people in your circle, it's best to steer the conversation in your favor, limit the time you spend together, or just avoid them completely. I had to accept that Breast Cancer is something that only those who have it, or survived it, could truly understand. So I had to lower my expectations of others and not allow their words to fester inside of me. So I accepted support and included a few people in certain parts of my treatment, but I kept my decisions and plans just between my immediate family. By doing this, I eliminated additional fears or stress from affecting me.

"Faith is taking the first
step even when you don't
see the whole staircase."

- Dr. Martin Luther King

{ notes }

Chapter 2

HELLO CHEMO

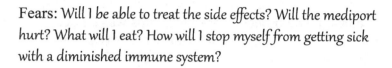

Fears: Will I be able to treat the side effects? Will the mediport hurt? What will I eat? How will I stop myself from getting sick with a diminished immune system?

The first part of my treatment consisted of 4 rounds of Chemotherapy. I would go to my oncologist every three weeks for Chemo for four hours. Learning that I had to go through Chemo destroyed my spirit. It literally broke me. The fear was overwhelming. I felt that it was completely unfair. At this point, I heard so many stories of people who had Breast Cancer treatment without Chemo and I was so angry that I was not one of them. I just couldn't fathom the idea of me being sick all the time or losing my hair! I had never been one to be sick and just be sick. I am usually the person who tries to shorten a cold or flu with home remedies, vitamins, and herbs. But for the first time in my life, I would have to just deal with it. I truly believe that it was during Chemo where I first started to truly apply my mantra, I would always tell myself you can cry and completely fall out today, but tomorrow, you are going to get up, adjust and fight! So I did just that and it helped me along the way.

Will I be able to treat the side effects? What will I eat? How will I stop myself from getting sick?

My first night of chemo was disastrous. I had no idea what I was doing. Although, I did all my research. I didn't know what to expect. After Chemo, I only felt a bit groggy and tired, so I assumed I was okay. I decided to eat pasta with chicken and broccoli for dinner- this was a huge mistake. I had the longest night of my life. My stomach was in knots and I was extremely constipated. It went on for hours. After that night, I did ample research on Chemo and I found out what I needed to do to ease my experience. I had my Chemo down to a science. Chemo stays in your system for 48 hours. So, I created a strategy that helped me get through it. Since I knew that the faster you flushed out the Chemo, the better you would feel, I created an effective strategy to flush the Chemo out of my system. I created a Chemo toolkit that I stuck to no matter what. I didn't consume any heavy foods during the first 4 days of chemo. My diet would mainly consist of the following:

Plums
Apples
Diced pear cups
Prune juice
Diced pears
Carrots
Broccoli
Kale salads
Naked smoothie
Sujo drinks
Frozen spinach/ kale
Wheat bread
Oatmeal

Granola bars
Pomegranate juice
Turkey soup
Soursop

First day:

For breakfast I would drink 2 cups of water and
1 green kale juice. I would eat an apple and a granola bar.

During my Chemo session

I would drink 12 cups of water. I would bring 6 bottles
and drink the rest from the water cooler. I would drink 1
berry smoothie, 1 green juice/smoothie, 2 cups of veggie
juice, 1 Soursop juice, and an 8 oz bottle of Pomegranate
juice.

After my Chemo session

I would go home and use my rebounder (mini-trampo-
line). By jumping on the trampoline I was able to flush out
the Chemo. It is known that a trampoline can help drain
your lymphatic system. Jumping on the trampoline boosts
your white blood cells. I would do this for 5 minutes or
until I got too tired.

I would also walk on the treadmill or outside. I would still
continue to consume more water.

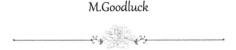

For dinner

I would drink a berry smoothie and eat either a kale salad or turkey soup with veggies. Turkey is a great thing to add to your diet. Turkey has Zinc in it and Zinc is known to boost your immune system. I would again consume more water.

After dinner

I would take an Epsom salt bath for 40 minutes. Epsom salt is great for detoxing. It will help you to remove the Chemo from your body faster. To get the full effect, you have to stay in for forty minutes. The first 20 minutes is to remove toxins and the last 20 minutes are to put the magnesium from the Epsom salt back into your body.

Since Chemo causes extremely painful gas and constipation, I would take Miralax mixed with Pomegranate juice as well as Dulcoease for gas

Second day

I would complete the same exact steps as on day one, but then I added other things to eat. Since Chemo symptoms pretty much change everyday, I had to add more remedies to help ease my experience.

So to avoid dry mouth, I would eat lemon drops, ice cream, sherbet, and popsicles.

I also begin to take the following vitamins:

> Turmeric
> Echinacea
> Apegenin
> Spirulina
> Vitamin D
> B12
> Vitamin E
> Coq10
> Zinc

These vitamins aren't proven to cure cancer, they are believed to help your immune system fight the cancer. For me, I took these vitamins to gain a bit of control in a sense. By using certain vitamins to prevent certain side effects, it made me feel as if I was helping myself. It gave me more trust in my treatment.

Third & fourth day

same food regimen as day 2, add 4 cups of green tea

I highlighted the four days because it usually takes four days until you feel the full effect of the Chemo, but in actuality, day 5-10 is typically when all side effects would come into play. During those days I kept the same diet. Once I started to feel as if I was out of the woods, I would

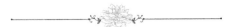

then add more of my normal food choices. I completed this plan for all 4 rounds of Chemo.

With Chemo, I found that exercise, acupuncture, meditation, and therapy were very helpful. It really takes more than just the physical to get through it. It takes mind control. There are times when you feel weak and want to give up, but if you win the mental battle, you can handle the physical.

Will 1 lose my hair?

The harsh reality of Chemo is that you will more than likely lose your hair. Many people think your hair falls out gradually, but no it falls out within two weeks of starting Chemo and no matter how much you prepare for it, you will still be in shock. For me, I decided to cut my hair right before the two week deadline. To my surprise it was already falling out. But by shaving my hair before hand, I didn't have to deal with the clunks of hair falling out. One thing that many people forget to tell you is that your hair will continue to fall out with every Chemo session. It will only start to grow once Chemo is completely finished. The good thing is my hair started to grow back a month after Chemo. So my advice to you is to consider purchasing wigs, scarfs, hats in advance. If you are prepared you will feel better. I believe that one of the things that helped me get through Chemo is my willingness to do whatever it takes to feel better. I felt that if I looked better I felt better. When I looked sick, I felt sick. So I made an effort to do things to make me feel beautiful or happy. So no matter how I felt, everyday I would get up and apply eyebrow makeup, eyeliner, mascara, and foundation. By doing this, it created a sense of normalcy. It's amazing what a little bit of makeup can do!

Will using a mediport hurt?

For me, the idea of getting a mediport was so frightening. I couldn't get used to the idea of having something protruding out of my skin. The thought of a nurse sticking a needle into the port made me cringe. Luckily my mediport experiences weren't too bad, because I learned early on the benefits of honesty and transparency when dealing with your doctor. With my doctors, I was never afraid to ask questions or express my true feelings. If I had a pet peeve, fear, or concern, I would share it with them. In sharing my complete fear of a nurse consistently accessing a mediport, I was blessed with a nurse who understood my fear and wanted to ease my pain. My nurse wrote me a prescription for Lidocaine. A clump of Lidocaine placed on top of your mediport, prevents pain. So on my Chemo day, I would liberally apply Lidocaine to the port and wrap it up in Saran Wrap, one hour before my appointment. By doing this, I eliminated any possibility of pain when the nurse inserted the IV inside of the port. One thing to remember about the port is, it's not as bad as it looks.

"You may not control all
the events that happen
to you, but you can decide
not to be reduced by them."

- Maya Angelou

{ notes }

Chapter 3

GOODBYE BOOBIES

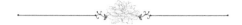

Fears: *Will people notice? Will I lose my mind? What do I need? How can I hide it? Will it hurt?*

Mastectomy is an amputation. It's the best way to explain it. No need to sugar coat it! It is an amputation, a removal of your breast, and just like any amputation it comes with side effects such as depression, shooting nerve pain, phantom pain, and numbness. I feel that it is one of the most brutal procedures a woman will take to save her life. Although, we frequently hear of people getting a mastectomy, we should never forget how traumatic it is to women.

After I completed my chemo, I was scheduled for a mastectomy. My mastectomy plan consisted of a bilateral mastectomy, then expanders for a couple of months, and then the exchange of expanders for implants. Fortunately, for me I was more than ready to have my breasts removed. It was amazing to me how initially the thought of a mastectomy was terrifying but after the difficult journey of Chemo, I felt that I was more than ready to take on whatever I needed to. I still had fears in regards to the mastectomy, but I felt an instant detachment towards my breasts. It was almost as if I hated them and no longer needed them. To me, they represented disease and I wanted all disease to be gone.

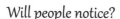

Will people notice?

One of the things you will notice right away as a Breast Cancer survivor is that as soon as you get surgery, everyone will stare. Everyone will look at you and wonder does she have breasts? Are those implants? It will be on everyone's mind for a while. One thing that concerned me was not knowing what I would wear to mask the lack of breasts. For my mastectomy, my doctor placed in expanders during surgery. Expanders are literally like balloons that are placed inside of your breasts. The doctor fills them up gradually until you've reached the breast size you both can agree on. They are pretty cool because they allow you to see beforehand, how you will look with your new breasts. One thing I learned right away, is that when it comes to a mastectomy, button-up shirts are your best friend. So in order to mask my breasts, I wore button-up shirts and scarves. It completely covered the breast area.

What do I need?

Knowing that I would be vulnerable during my recovery, I was determined to be over-prepared for my surgery. To ease my anxiety, I washed and braided my hair in advance, bought all button-up clothes, set up a table on the side of my bed for meds, and bought a bed desk for eating. I can honestly say I needed all these items! I was over-prepared and it paid off. In order to ensure that your mastectomy will go smoother, you will need the following items:

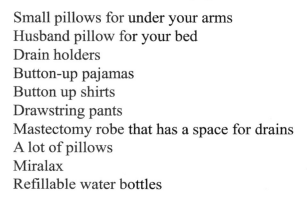

Small pillows for under your arms
Husband pillow for your bed
Drain holders
Button-up pajamas
Button up shirts
Drawstring pants
Mastectomy robe that has a space for drains
A lot of pillows
Miralax
Refillable water bottles

Before your surgery, be sure to have plans for the following:

Either cook and freeze meals for at least two weeks or find someone who is willing to cook or coordinate your meals for two weeks. Thoroughly clean your home in advance, it will be hard to clean your home for a while. If you are a parent or pet owner, find someone who is willing to help you care for your kids or pets. Contact your kid's school, inform them of your surgery. Coordinate carpooling with your family and friends.

Will I lose my mind?

My biggest fear was that I would lose my mind once I woke up without my breasts. I was frightened by this. I stayed up for nights trying to imagine how I could mentally prepare for the first time I saw my breast after surgery. I came up with so many ideas to avoid seeing them. I wanted to place sheets over the mirrors in the bathroom, I wanted to place sheets over the mirrors in the bathroom, I wanted to hide my breast area from my husband, I was so determined to not see my breasts until they were filled up by the expanders. In my mind, I just knew that the moment I saw my breasts, I would crumble and lose my will to fight. After going crazy about this for months, I started to research online how other women who have had this procedure looked after surgery. Research eased my fears by preparing me for what I might see. I knew that a mastectomy procedure would be more of a mental battle than a physical one. So I got myself ready to fight.

Everyday, I would literally talk to myself. I told myself that no matter what it looked like it was temporary and I would not allow it to destroy me. I told myself consistently, that you are saving your life, no matter the outcome, you will make the best of it. You will find a way to get it through it. Surprisingly, this worked! Although, I was still in disbelief when I first saw my breasts after surgery, I didn't lose my mind. I accepted that this would be a mental challenge and I refused to lose it. So, I told myself, you are going through a transition, it's not over yet, but the best part about it, is you are now Cancer free.

Will it hurt?

I will say that a mastectomy is a huge undertaking. It's draining and just alot to physically and mentally take on. Since you can't raise your arms for two weeks or sleep on your side, sleeping comfortably is difficult. You will need help. I needed help to shower and move around. You have to rest. I didn't experience too much pain due to the fact that I felt sedated most of the time. I took my meds around the clock. I also, gave myself time to rest and relax. However, the one thing I hated the most were the drains. I found the drains to be scary, disgusting, and hurtful. I could not wait to have them removed. However, I did find my drain holder to be very effective in helping me to keep the drain in one place and limiting the pain. For me the mental pain associated with the mastectomy was more difficult than the physical pain. I hated the fact that I needed help to shower, get dressed, change my drains, and etc. Although I welcomed the help, I was hurt more by the fact that I couldn't hide my chest, and my caregiver, who was my husband had to see it. It was a lot to accept and take in initially. But as the shock wore off and the days went by, I became more comfortable with my chest and the help that I was receiving . I believe that I was able to adjust because I was prepared. The following items helped me get through my mastectomy.

Things you should do before surgery:

Purchase all mastectomy garments
Place everything you may need within reach
Purchase a seat belt pillow
Get waxed
Shampoo hair
Pedicure/ manicure
Place all snacks on lower cabinet
Buy button up blouses & pajamas

Set up table on side of bed
Buy books and magazines
Buy husband pillow
Small pillows to place under arm
Battery operated toothbrush
Wipes
Spray deodorant
Use pill dispenser
Notebook to monitor drains
Select a person to keep notes of all doctor info
Find helpful organizations that help with bills, cleaning
service, pet sitters, etc.

Day of surgery

Pajamas that button up in the front
Pants with a drawstring
Drained carrier
Chapstick

For home:

Side table placed next to my bed for medicine, vitamin
and drinks
Food tray for the bed
Husband pillow
Button pajamas
Pillow for under my arm
Soft mastectomy bra that opened to the front
24hr hot/cold cup

To go outside:

Shirts that button up
Scarfs that could disguise lack of breast
Drain carrier

"We delight in the beauty of
the butterfly, but rarely
admit the changes it has gone
through to achieve that beauty."

- Maya Angelou

{ notes }

Chapter 4

NEW BOOBS

Fears: *Will the expanders hurt? How can I live without sensation? Will I be able to hug my kids?*

Will expanders hurt ?

I loved my expanders! I felt they gave me life and it was not because they were beautiful or comfortable, it was because I was starting to feel normal. Don't get me wrong expanders are hard and uncomfortable, they actually suck, but they are great at helping you to see what your future breasts may look like. Because I had to get my expanders filled, I was only truly without the appearance of breasts for two weeks. After two weeks, my doctor would insert a needle into the expander, which didn't hurt at all, the insertion looks worse than it feels. So the doctor would fill them up little by little until they are a good size for my body. It took about two months to get them completely filled. During that time, I felt completely uncomfortable and anxious. The expanders were tight and felt like a hard ball. It was hard to get used to. After they were filled, I had an exchange surgery. This surgery was short, about an hour long and way easier than a mastectomy.

How can I live without sensation?

When I found out about my diagnosis, it was easy for me to choose a mastectomy because I knew my strengths and

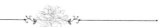

weaknesses and I knew what I could live with and also I knew it was necessary to prolong my life. But one of the things I feared the most is the loss of sensation. To lose the ability to feel anything, truly hurt my soul. It felt like a loss, felt like I was in someone else's body. Depending on the weather, implants can be very cold. They are uncomfortable, hard, and you may experience phantom pain. All those side effects bothered me truly, but what bothered me most is my complete disconnect from my breasts. My breasts truly just became a cosmetic necessity. They serve no purpose, other than to make me feel whole. To be honest, the loss of sensation still is something I struggle with. It's something that affects me randomly and makes me sad. However, these past two years have helped me to realize that sensation is a small price to pay when it comes to extending your life. By appreciating the fact that I was fortunate enough to get a nipple sparing mastectomy and fortunate enough to have minimal unexpected issues, I am becoming more comfortable with my new breasts. I am learning to live with the new me. Although my breasts feel foreign to my body, I am happy to have them.

Will I be able to hug my kids?

Before my exchange, I read somewhere that you will never hug your kids the same. That bothered me deeply. It overwhelmed me completely. I just felt like I lost and gave up so much, that I couldn't possibly survive without their hugs. Fortunately, I still hug my kids like crazy and I still feel the love. However, after getting new breasts, I hate to hug adults. I barely hug friends or family and it's not always think that they can feel my implants. But I realize this feeling is in my mind and is stupid. It's my life, I had Cancer, had to have a mastectomy and now I just have to learn to love the new me.

"My mission in life is not merely to survive, but to thrive; and to do so with some passion, some compassion, some humor, and some style."

- Maya Angelou

{ notes }

Chapter 5

RADIATION SUCKS

Fears: *Will my skin return back to normal?*

Radiation

Just when I thought the hard part was behind me, I was scheduled for 5 weeks of radiation. 5 weeks of radiation translates to 25 sessions, which is 25 days. Same time every day for a month. In my mind radiation was scary, but I had no idea what to expect. I had gotten used to a little bit of normalcy. Since I had already had my Chemo, mastectomy, and expander exchange, I felt ready and willing to take on the world. I felt like I had gotten some parts of my life back. However, I was so wrong...radiation was a struggle for me. I found the most difficult part of radiation was going to a radiation session daily for 5 weeks. Although the sessions were quick and painless, going there every day was mentally draining. It felt as if I was tricked into thinking that the worst part was behind me, but completely unprepared for the final part of the journey that lied ahead.

As the radiation progressed, my skin started to burn badly. Within my third week of radiation, my skin began to break. It remained wet and oozy. This was completely devastating. I literally felt as if I had hit my breaking point. It felt like all my hard work through this Cancer journey was all for nothing. I had just gotten my new boobs, and radiation was damaging my left breast with each session. My breasts began to look charred. The nipples were fading and the breasts were oozing. It was a nightmare that actually got worse after the sessions ended. I was in so much pain, that I had to get a prescription, just to stop the pain. This completely depressed me. I just felt like I couldn't win. My biggest fear was that my skin would never return to it's original color. I didn't believe that it would heal. It was difficult to imagine that this much damage could be fixed. After about a month after radiation, my breasts started to heal. Surprisingly, my broken skin healed and the pain stopped. My remained a bit tinted but everything was pretty much back to normal. Each month after treatment, it got better and better.

What to use for your radiation burns?

During my treatment, I learned very quickly that I could not control or prevent burns, but I could manage them and make sure that I was comfortable. So it became my goal, to use creams and home remedies, that made the burns more bearable. Here are some remedies that helped me during radiation:

• Wear button up shirts to treatment, something soft and flowy.

• As soon as you start treatment, before there are any signs of burning, apply the aloe vera plant liberally throughout the day immediately after treatment and continuously.

• Before you go to treatment, be sure to not wear any

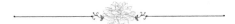
creams or deodorants, wearing the wrong thing can contribute to burning.

• Calendula oil and Tamanu oil are great for healing. Apply them consistently.

• Use aquaphor.

• If skins starts to break, use a thick layer of silvadene.

• Never be afraid to discuss the burn with your doctors, they have some prescriptions meds and creams that can help you with the burn.

• Saline soaks are very helpful. Take a paper towel, soak it in saline, and lay it over your burn.

• Placing your cream in the freezer can feel like heaven. It's a perfect way to cool off the burn.

• Since my burns, were similar to a horrible baby rash. I found that Desitin was very effective in helping to heal my skin.

What can I do to help my skin?

Aside from using the correct creams, one thing you can do to help your skin heal is physical therapy. I know this may sound strange to some. It most definitely sounded strange to me, but it really works. After my skin healed, I started physical therapy. I went weekly. My physical

therapist would help me perform certain exercises to help my arm and skin. Since radiation is drying, it can cause your lymph nodes to dry out and tighten. It can also affect the elasticity in your skin, which could make your arm hard to lift. So the physical therapy helps to keep your arm moving and to massage out scar tissue. It's a very effective part of treatment. I still go to physical therapy weekly.

"Cause I think we can make it, in fact, I'm sure ......
And if you fall, stand tall and come back for more."

-Tupac

{ notes }

Chapter 6

WHAT ABOUT YOUR FRIENDS?

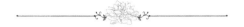

Fears: How will I deal with relatives & friends who have completely neglected/forgotten about me?

In this journey, there are gifts along the way-this is what I learned during my Breast Cancer journey. Every negative situation that occurred, bought positivity to light. In my journey, the greatest gift I received was the revealing of friendships. As soon as I was diagnosed, I immediately lost friends. For most people the thought of losing life long friendships while you are sick, just doesn't make sense. But in the Breast Cancer journey, it is way too common. That college friend who you spoke to every day, that friend who you always had their back, the first cousin who you helped get into college, or that cousin who you supported through every endeavor or event, may all abandon you in your time of need. They will claim "you didn't look sick" or " I didn't know how to help" or " you were secretive". There will be a million excuses for not simply calling to say "hello"or "how are you doing?". No matter what their excuses are, graciously let them go. Let them go without wonder, without resentment, or without anger. Because the reality is, more than likely that relationship was one sided, draining, time consuming, financially consuming and just an additional stress you don't need. These relationships themselves, may have been a Cancer, you needed to cut out.

In my experience, you lose who you needed to lose and you gained those who you needed to win. While I lost some friendships that I thought were valuable, I gain some friendships that were magical! I gained truly unexpected friendships. People who simply became my friend out of concern. People who devoted their time to help with my errands, sat with my husband through my surgeries, took my kids out for ice cream just so they could get away, bought me protein shakes and smoothies, planned a brunch to get me ready for chemo, hosted a fundraiser to help me with expenses, made me soup and brownies, and those who just texted funny memes or words of encouragement-these were my true friends. Everyday people that I considered to be an ex classmate, colleague, or associate came through and was there for me during the scariest moments of my life.

In the past two years, I have created bonds with classmates from grade school to women in other countries going through my same journey. I learned the true meaning of friendship during this journey. It's not who could afford to buy stuff or show up, it's who carved out time in their life to think of me. Whether it was a card or a text, just the fact that they thought of me, meant the most to me. However, I do understand that Breast Cancer is scary to close relatives or friends, but a hello or wellness check is easy to do. There is no excuse. The beauty of Breast Cancer is that it gave me insight. I was doing too much for the wrong people. I was too invested in their lives and they didn't return the favor. So I let them go without anger, but what I learned through it all, is perspective.

Breast Cancer gave me the beauty of revealing friend-ships. Although I lost some friends and close family members, I embrace that our season together has ended and that's ok. With the help of my new and improved support system, I am more prepared and motivated to fight. Because of them, I have never felt alone and I am forever grateful

Do I need to network with other survivors?

Whether it is in a support group, forum, or via social media, you should most definitely network with survivors. Survivors are crucial to your success! They are the best resource out there. I have learned so much just by connecting with other Breast Cancer patients and survivors. I have learned how to fight, live, be positive, and push through. Your family and friends, although they may mean well, they truly have no idea of what you are going through. They are new to this journey and don't know what to expect. Some of my fears, concerns, or questions that I had at 2 am in the morning, have been answered by survivors. When you doctor is unavailable, you can gain a little hope and inspiration from someone who has been there. As a Breast Cancer Patient, it can be so difficult to make decisions that is in your best interest. It's hard to be your own advocate, but by connecting with other Breast Cancer patients/survivors, sometimes they can direct you and tell you the questions you should be asking. They can pinpoint areas where staff or doctors maybe lacking. They can provide insight and advice that is proven to work. Being a survivor gives you firsthand knowledge of the

Breast Cancer journey. I believe that they are a great resource and the key to your success. There is nothing more uplifting than to meet women who have your same diagnosis.

During my journey, I created an online platform via Instagram. This allowed me to globally connect with Breast Cancer survivors. This connection has been rewarding and truly feeds my soul. There are so many women sharing their journey on social media platforms. These women are bringing awareness and hope. Here are some of my favorite places to connect with other Breast Cancer survivors online:

Young Black Women Fighting & Surviving Breast Cancer Facebook Group

Young Survival Coalition Facebook Group

For the breast of us blog

Shay Sharpe's Pink Wishes

Breast Cancer Healthline

Living Beyond Breast Cancer

My Cancer Chic

Cancer at Thirty

"The most common
way people give up their
power is by thinking
they don't have any."

- Alice Walker

{ notes }

Chapter 7

NEW NORMAL

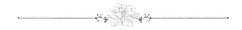

Fears: 1 will never get my life back? How will 1 manage my day to day?

At some point in this journey, it will start to feel as if you will never get your life back. Even when you think you got back in the swing of things, something will happen to make you feel as if you will never have normalcy. Unfortunately, this is the beast of this journey. No matter how far you may come, there maybe setbacks and issues that make you feel as if you will never get your life back. But what I have come to realize, things will start to feel normal. It will be a new normal. You won't get your life back exactly how it was, but you can create a new life that is more meaningful, humble, and passionate. A life that simply takes the time to smell the roses and enjoy the sun.

For me, I look at life after Cancer, as a clean slate. All the fears or issues I had before Cancer seem irrelevant. I learned to value my time and to spend time wisely. To spend it free from fear or anger. Before Cancer I lived a very cautious life, fearful of taking risks. Now I understand how precious life is and how precious my time is, so I strive to live a life that is more adventurous and fun. A more meaningful life. In doing so, I search for things to enrich my life. I made a bucket list and actually completed the items on my list. I share my story with other women who need inspiration, I believe in building sisterhood and

How to manage day to day?

It can be very difficult to get through your day without fear. I get through my day to day by focusing on the things that I can control. I can control what I eat, so I eat well. I can control what I see, so I stay away from things that make me sad. I stopped googling Cancer issues and focused more on things that make me smile. This journey helped me discover myself. It helped me find what made me happy. So I get through each day surrounded by things that make me smile. I am very careful of what I allow to get into my space. I control my space as best as I can. So I don't tolerate negativity from others. I strive every single day to create internal happiness. It's not easy and some days it's quite difficult but it is a goal I make for myself.

In my journey for peace, health, and sanity, I am always in search of ways to help defeat this disease and keep me happy. As a way to relieve my mind of stress, I did two things: one, I wrote a book called " BK's mother has Breast Cancer", a children's book to help children understand and deal with their mother's Breast Cancer diagnosis. This book helped me to gain control of my mental state by writing a book that could help others. It made me feel as if I was still being a problem solver. Two, I started playing Angry birds on my phone. I know this sounds silly, but it is one of my biggest stress relievers. Although, I was familiar with the game and played years ago, I never really got into it. But in this journey, it has been my saving grace! Whenever, I am overwhelmed, I will play this game for hours, it completely relaxes me and changes my mental state. It literally puts me at peace and makes me happy. Whatever I was just worrying about, I forget instantly once I become engulfed into the game. I will play anywhere! In the doctor's office before appointments, late at night when I get overcome with fear, or just anytime when I need to refocus or forget. By playing Angry Birds consistently, I learned a valuable lesson in this journey, I learned to do whatever you need to do to keep your peace and to survive.

How to live with fatigue?

One thing that is too familiar to most Cancer survivors is fatigue. Fatigue is an ongoing struggle. For me, it started when I was on Chemo and just continued throughout my entire journey. I now deal with it with my hormone replacement therapy meds. I have found that fatigue is not preventable. It definitely gets in the way of living day to day. In order to gain some control, I try to exercise, read, or work in the very beginning of the day. Since I know that my body essentially gives out in the afternoon, I try to complete most of my difficult tasks of the day early. If I am at home and feel fatigue, I embrace it. I slow down and relax. But when I can't embrace the fatigue, I find that pushing through can be very helpful. When I stay busy and focus on something else, I can push through.

Holistic Healing

Aside from my traditional treatment and meds, I am an avid believer in holistic healing. This belief strengthened during my Cancer journey. I actually believe in applying all things and seeing what works. So I am pretty flexible in my treatment plan. I am open to the traditional route as well as the holistic. Since I take Tamoxifen daily and a Zoladex shot monthly, there are so many side effects and unwanted symptoms from this combination. I struggle with sleeping and hot flashes. One of the things I do to combat these symptoms is acupuncture. I go for acupuncture session twice a month. These sessions have been not only helpful in helping me to sleep well and have less hot flashes, but also it has helped to regain movement in my arm where some of my lymph nodes have been removed. I also enjoy yoga. Yoga has been very helpful in creating a space where I can relax and unwind. The stretching movements have helped me strengthen the movement in my arm. Not to mention yoga was very easy for me to do continuously while going through treatment. I believe that in order to heal your body, you must also heal your mind. So, I meditate daily more than once a day. I take time to breathe correctly and relax my mind. I find it to be so relaxing and beneficial to my body.

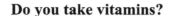

Do you take vitamins?

I have found that in this journey, I feel the most powerful when I feel that I am contributing to my health. I don't like to just rely on traditional medicine. I like to explore herbs, spices,certain foods, and vitamins. With the proper research and approval from your doctor, you can add so many vitamins to help you on your journey.

Here are a list of the vitamins I have added to my regimen.

Turmeric

Spirulina

Mushrooms

Apegenin

Black Seed Oil

Magnesium

Melatonin

Valerian Root

Vitamin D

Hair Loss

As with everything, time is your friend. This is definitely the case with hair loss. For me, my hair started to grow right after chemo. However, certain areas of my hair remained lighter. My eyebrows and eyelashes have remained very faint and thin. They have not fully recovered yet. In order to promote growth, I use the following:

• Castor oil

• Vitamin E

• Rogaine

One of the things I learned most about Breast Cancer is the art of redirecting or enhancing. As my hair struggled to come back, instead of crying I used that time to experiment with fun creative styles and colors.

Weight Gain

During the Cancer journey, it can be difficult to lose weight. Ever since I started treatment, my weight continues to fluctuate up and down. Different procedures and medicines contribute to weight gain. It's completely frustrating! It can feel like you are fighting a losing battle. I would literally be working out and not losing weight! One of the things that has helped me to lose weight is intermittent fasting. Intermittent fasting is basically changing your eating patterns. By eating and fasting on a strict

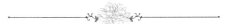

schedule, you can lose weight. During the fasting period, your cells are replenished.To lose weight, I fast for 16 hours and then I only eat for 8 hours. I basically eat from 12pm - 8pm, then I fast from 8pm - 11am. Here are some of the benefits of intermittent fasting:

Weight loss

Lower risk of type 2 diabetes

Improved heart health

Improved brain health

Reduced risk of cancer

Boost metabolism

May slow down aging process

Hormone Replacement Therapy

As part of my post Breast Cancer treatment, the doctors prescribed hormone replacement therapy. This means that I take a Tamoxifen pill daily for 5-10 years. Since my Breast Cancer was Estrogen Receptive, the Tamoxifen helps to prevent reoccurrence. As with every drug, there are many side effects associated with Tamoxifen. I have been taking Tamoxifen for over a year now and luckily, the only side effects that I have experienced are weight gain and hot flashes. Of course, these are not ideal side effects. But through this journey, I have learned to be grateful and refocus. I know first hand that it can always be worse. Taking a pill daily is no fun, but I tell myself that it's helping me to fight the battles I can't fight on my own. I know that many women quit their Tamoxifen and I completely understand. It would definitely be much easier to live a life free of side effects and the threat of Uterine Cancer, which is a rare side effect of Tamoxifen. There are times, that I, myself wanted to quit. But I decided to fight and give it a try. I have decided to be open minded and try anything that may save my life. I believe that there isn't one way to beat Cancer. It will take many different combinations of meds, fruits, herbs, vegetables, and holistic healing. I believe that with this mindset, I can make it to year five or year ten on Tamoxifen.

Depression

During this journey, you are on a constant emotional roller coaster. You are bombarded with so much information and fear, it can be difficult to process. Depression can seep in before treatment, during treatment, and after treatment. For me, I experienced bits of depression throughout my journey. Every time I had to do a new procedure or take new meds, it would send my body in an uproar. I initially lived in a constant state of fear. Until one day, I realized that a lot of my fear was triggered by three things: my meds, browsing cancer information online, and worrying about my future. Once I recognized my triggers, I was able to help myself. Whenever I started to feel overwhelmed, I would meditate to release stress. I stopped

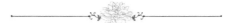

googling medical terminology online and I backed away from Breast Cancer forums from time to time. I made a constant effort to control what I saw or felt. So I started doing things that made me happy. I refused to engage in trivial things that bought drama. I just felt that my first battle with Breast Cancer, would be a battle to keep my sanity and happiness. So, I always fought to find a way to relax my mind and make me feel better. I am a firm believer of anti-depressants. Before Cancer, I never really thought about anti-depressants, but after Cancer, I definitely believe that it is sometimes needed to combat the depressing side effects of some meds. Breast Cancer survivors have to fight all the time, we can use all the help that is available to us. I am also a firm believer in holistic healing. To combat my depression, I started acupuncture. Acupuncture has helped me tremendously. After treatment, I feel relaxed, I sleep better, and feel happier.

"Living in the moment means letting go of the past and not waiting for the future. It means living your life consciously, aware that each moment you breathe is a gift."

— Oprah Winfrey

{ notes }

Chapter 8

TERMS TO KNOW & RESOURCES

Support Groups, Online Platforms and Organizations

Many times I meet women who have been newly diagnosed and they are always surprised about the wealth of knowledge that I have acquired in such a short time. They have yet to realize that my level of knowledge about the Breast Cancer journey is from experience and basically researching every aspect of this disease whenever I had the chance. The best way to gain trusted information is through Breast Cancer support groups and organizations. These groups can quickly get you up to speed and prepare you for what's to come. Since I live in the DC area, some of my groups are local to me. But, you can find local and national groups to help you on your journey. Here is a list of some of the groups and organizations I used to help me on my journey:

Young Survival Coalition Facebook Group:
An online platform that allows you to meet and connect with young Breast Cancer patients and survivors.

For the Breast of Us:
An online Breast Cancer community for young women of color.

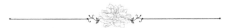

The Breasties:
A non profit organization dedicated to supporting young women affected by breast and reproductive cancers through community and friendship.

Breast Cancer Healthline App:
A social community support chat where Breast Cancer patients can connect with other Breast Cancer patients.

Living Beyond Breast Cancer:
A nonprofit organization providing trusted information and a community of support to all impacted by Breast Cancer.

Blossoming Butterfly:
A nonprofit organization dedicated to providing emotional and financial support to families who are out of work due to their battle with Breast Cancer.

Shay Sharpe's Pink Wishes:
A nonprofit organization that educates, advocates, and grants wishes to young women affected by Breast Cancer.

Young Black Women Fighting & Surviving Breast Cancer Facebook Group
Created by Breast Cancer Survivor, Marquita Goodluck. A support group for young women of color who have been affected by Breast Cancer. A place where fighters, thrivers, and survivors can connect, share experiences, get informed, and support.

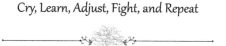
Tigerlily Foundation:
A non profit organization whose mission is to educate, advocate, support, and empower young women with Breast Cancer.

Charge Up Campaign:
A nonprofit organization supporting cancer survivors and caregivers faced with health, social, and economic issues.

Cleaning for a Reason:
A nonprofit organization that gives the gift of free house cleaning to women undergoing treatment for any type of cancer.

Breastcancer.org:
A nonprofit organization dedicated to providing information and community to those touched by Breast Cancer.

Sisters Network:
A nonprofit organization committed to increasing national attention to the devastating impact that Breast Cancer has in the African American community.

Terms to know: Toxins to Avoid

A Breast Cancer diagnosis will require so many changes, the biggest change for me, was the items that I purchased. Many of our everyday products that we use are filled with toxins. Everything from shampoo to makeup. For this reason, I am more mindful of the beauty products that I purchase for myself and my family. I take the time to understand and learn about the ingredients that I put on my skin. Although, I know that it can be difficult to avoid everything, my goal is to drastically limit my exposure to such toxins. Here is a list of some toxins I try to avoid:

• **Paraben:**
(isobutylparaben, butylparaben, methylparaben, propylparaben)

Preservatives found in some makeup, deodorant, sunscreen, lotions, hair products and personal care items. Known to mimic estrogen and increase the risk of Breast Cancer.

• **Formaldehyde**
(DMDM Hydantoin, Imidazolidinyl urea, Diazolidinyl urea, Quaternium-15, Bronopol, Hydroxymethylglycinate)

A proven carcinogen found in nail polish, shampoo, bodywash, and eyelash glue.

• **Phthalates**
(phthalates dibutyl phthalate, dimethyl phthalate, diethyl phthalate)

Known to be a carcinogen. Found in nail polishes, perfumes, soaps, and shampoos.

My Shopping List

In my opinion, the best thing you can do for yourself in this journey is to control the controllables. Since a Breast Cancer diagnosis brings such a powerless feeling, I have found that there is power in taking control of your nutrition and health. I find that by paying close attention to the foods I consume, I gain more control. I always feel as if I am fighting Cancer from all angles. With so much research, I have created a consistent grocery list that I feel has been helpful to my recovery and happiness. Here is a typical list of the groceries I buy weekly:

Fruits & Vegetables:

Blueberries
Strawberries
Raspberries
Mushrooms
Pineapples
Broccoli
Garlic

Tomatoes
Green and red peppers
Olives
Onions

Drinks:

Pomegranate juice
Soursop juice
Green tea
Turmeric tea
Alkaline water
Kombucha

Meats:

Salmon
Tuna

Oil:

Olive oil
Coconut oil

"It's not the load that breaks you down, it's the way you carry it."

— Lena Horne

{ notes }

Chapter 9

PAY IT FORWARD

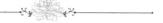

Ways you can help

How others helped me

Sisterhood

The unfortunate gift of Breast Cancer, is the beauty of sisterhood. The bonds created through this horrible disease are simply magical. From the moment I received my diagnosis, Breast Cancer survivors stepped in and were there to help. I have met some amazing women who have guided me and counseled me along the way. Whether I had a fear or concern, they were there to give me perspective. Since a Breast Cancer diagnosis can be so lonely, it was refreshing to gain insight and friendship from survivors. Their support gave me hope. By just simply sharing their journey, gave me the strength and courage to fight through my journey. Because of them, I knew what to expect before procedures, I knew how to deal with my children, and I knew where to find much needed resources.

Once I completed my treatment, I began to return the favor. Over the past two years, I have helped women as they began their journey. Whether it is a monthly phone conversation, connecting online, or sharing information. I devote my time to sharing my experience with others. I plan to always take time to help others in need. I wrote a children's book, entitled " BK's Mommy Has Breast Cancer" to help women and their children deal with their Breast Cancer diagnosis.

Because of my experience, I believe that once you are healed, it is essential that every Breast Cancer survivor pay it forward. Whether it is a conversation or simply passing a book along, it is important that we connect with others and share our experiences. By sharing our experience, we can save lives. It is important hat we are honest and vulnerable enough to show others the way. A big part of beating this disease is your frame of mind. Positivity will get you far. It can be difficult to be positive when you are facing so many obstacles. By simply befriending a Breast Cancer survivor, you give them a reason to fight. You are an example they can strive to be. Although, I had support from family and friends, I will forever be grateful for the support and friendship I received from women I only bonded with due to this horrible disease.

Here are some of the ways you can help others:

Be a friend
Attend appointments
Send a monthly card
Share your experience
Cook meals
Walk with them
Make them laugh
Be open to chat freely
Create an online platform and share your experience

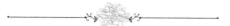

Open door policy
Make a gift basket
Order food
Give them questions to ask doctors
Refer great doctors
Regift Breast Cancer products you no longer need

"You may encounter many defeats, but you must not be defeated. In fact, it may be necessary to encounter the defeats, so you can know who you are, what you can rise from, how you can still come out of it."

— Maya Angelou

{ notes }

Chapter 10

SURVIVING & THRIVING

Fears: *How will I love the new me? How will I make it to year 10?*

Loving yourself is an arduous task. It is one of the hardest things you will be forced to do in this journey. Every time you think you are strong, you will be challenged many times over. Dealing with your new normal will be a challenge. It will be a constant battle. I believe it takes practice to learn to change your perspective. Perspective is the best thing you can have on this journey. You will not always be confident. There will be moments where you will have doubt but this is when you will most definitely need to apply my mantra, CRY, LEARN, ADJUST, FIGHT & REPEAT! Surviving Breast Cancer is difficult on many levels. It's a constant battle to stay positive and upbeat. With so many scars and a new normal, it can be difficult to embrace the changes in your life. What I have learned so far in this journey, is to look at the bigger picture always. To focus on the positive areas of my life. Although, a Breast Cancer journey can make your future seem dim and your days seem short. It is important that you never live this way. Never live life as if it is ending ,Instead live it as if it is beginning. Treasure every moment.

For me, I hated being vulnerable. I hated the change. I wanted nothing more than to have my old life back. I felt cheated. But what I have learned is that my life was great before, but it was flawed. I lived in fear. I lived for others

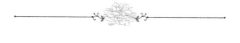

and I lived cautiously. Breast Cancer showed me my strength. If I could make the hard decisions that I have made thus far and live with the scars and an unpromising fate, I knew that I could accomplish anything I wanted. So I decided to live a life for me. One that was filled with adventure, more willing to try new things, and more meaningful. I made a bucket list of everything I wanted to accomplish in life and I work consistently to complete it. In my life, I practice self care, stay clear of toxic people, and toxic situations. In a weird way, Breast Cancer has set me free. It has allowed me to shape the life that I want. I am way more fearless. Of course, I have days when I get sad, worried, or can't seem to shake it. But, I embrace those days and always remember this feeling, this moment shall pass. I know that I am human and I have to allow myself to heal and experience all the emotions that come with this journey. So instead of fighting the bad moments, I go through it and I always, always remember to CRY, LEARN, ADJUST, FIGHT & REPEAT!

"I have learned over the years that when one's mind is made up, this diminishes fear; knowing what must be done does away with fear."

-Rosa Parks

{ notes }

CPSIA information can be obtained
at www.ICGtesting.com
Printed in the USA
BVHW041502211019
561663BV00010B/676/P